MEDITERRANEAN COOKBOOK FOR BEGINNERS

1000 CALORIES A DAY MEAL PLAN: HEALTHY LIFESTYLE EASY: DELICIOUS RECIPES: ULTIMATE DIET PLAN

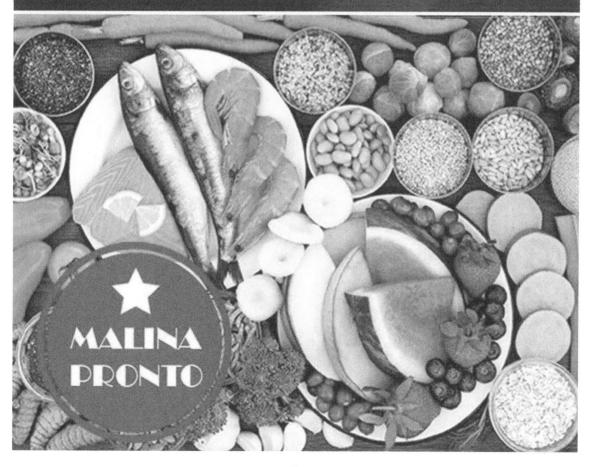

MALINA PRONTO

Mediterranean Diet Cookbook For Beginners 1000 Calories A Day Meal Plan: Healthy Lifestyle Easy: Delicious Recipes: Ultimate Diet Plan

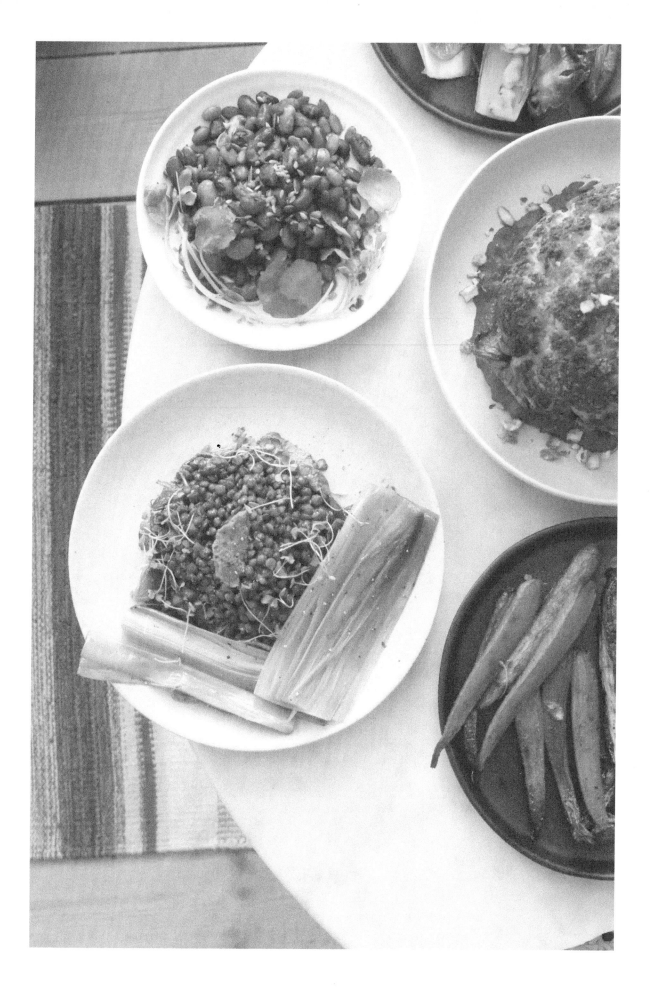

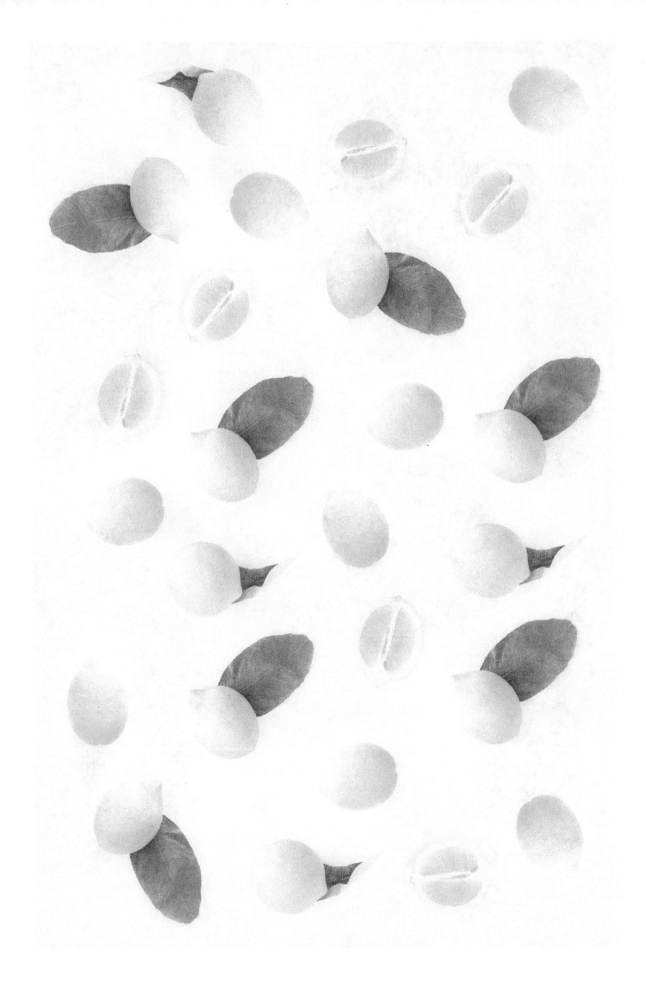

1. Mediterranean Diet Cookbook.

Various scientists have tracked down that standard Mediterranean menu is perhaps the most nutritious and best on earth - ideal for weight decrease and lower speeds of cardiovascular diseases and other steady conditions. The Mediterranean public have reliably liked the benefits of Mediterranean food sources by following plans that will captivate your feeling of taste, feed body and soul - and can be set up effectively in your home kitchen.

The amount of people who look for better eating regimens is building up every day, and enormous quantities of those people are searching for an ideal Mediterranean cookbook which would satisfy their necessities. Along these lines, Mediterranean eating routine dinner plans are growing in reputation, and anything is possible from that point and more cook books are being dispersed.

Mediterranean cooking is especially moving on new vegetables, natural items, fish, poultry and flavors. Various Mediterranean eating routine cookbooks advance direct, ordinary Mediterranean menus from Italy, Spain, southern France, Greece, Tunis and elsewhere. Most plans in Mediterranean eating routine cook books cut down on added fats, red meat and dairy things, highlight low to coordinate use of food assortments from animal sources (like lean meat, poultry and fish), anyway are rich in vegetables, natural items, vegetables, grains and other strong wellsprings of supplements and minerals.

Every Mediterranean eating routine cookbook highlights the usage of olive oil as the main fat which substitutes essentially any excess wellsprings of fats from animals and plants. Novice cooks as experienced ones will be energized through incidental and scrumptious Mediterranean plans well off in flavor and strong enhancements, yet low in drenched fats and cholesterol.

With plans bursting in flavor and sound enhancements, easy to prepare and made by extensive of results of the dirt, grains and vegetables, fish, lean meats, and brilliant desserts, various Mediterranean eating routine cookbooks are made for the current American kitchens.

In any of these Mediterranean eating routine cook books you'll similarly find new cooking strategies and an enhanced method to manage cooking which will surely fulfill everyone since straightforwardness is the thing that is the issue here.

Straightforwardness is the route in to the Mediterranean menu - essential trimmings and serene game plan and cooking. Mediterranean eating routine cookbooks are more than a cookbook - they are graphs for better living! Mediterranean eating routine plans have been carefully modified to present to you the most flawlessly awesome from the Mediterranean territory.

2. Top Delicious Recipes.

There are a couple of important methodology and how to tips to turn out sublime plans. Deglazing is one such huge methodology that can change a respectable tasting equation to an amazing tasting one.

Deglazing a skillet

The ensuing stage to sauteing is deglazing.

Exactly when you fry or saute trimmings a tanish remaining is left sticking to the compartment. It is the left over food particles in any case called loving. These particles are truly molded from the caramelization of trademark sugars of the trimmings being singed and contain a lot of concentrated flavor.

What you need to do is, take some liquid which is stock, wine or water and pour it to the dish. By then put the holder in a difficult spot on the glow and tenderly piece out these particles.

If the equation contains high proportion of fat, that can be coordinated with the use of acidic liquids to deglaze like lemon press and wines.

The liquid which has been added to the dish can be used multiplely.

First thing it might be re-added to the equation being cooked. Or on the other hand the flavor can be reinforced with the development of specific flavors and flavors to the liquid.

In fact, even flour can be added to make the mix thick. Or then all in all it might be used in the making of a sauce base.

Cooking techniques, for instance, deglazing are generally more notable with meat than vegetables.

Caramelizing

One more kind of singing cooperation which follows sauteing.

At the point when the holder trimmings turn clear by sauteing trimmings hold cooking to the point that they become natural hued. This draws out the typical agreeableness in food sources, and raises flavor and scent of the dish.

Other flavor redesigning tips are:

Toasting flavors and nuts conveyances their standard oil and brings out mind blowing flavor.

Moderate cooking is an uncommon strategy to improve flavor especially when making sauce or curry based plans, stews and soups.

Use margarine (prevalently western cooking) instead of oil, as it gives out more flavor on warming and improves designs to the extent that used unassumingly.

Another course is to use trimmings which supplement each other. If you find dull blended greens extreme, add some fat and destructive when warming, so the flavor advances down.

All of these tips and misleads can help in bettering cooking techniques, to deliver more superb plans.

3. Day Meal Plan.

You are overweight and wild eyed to lose some resolved pounds. You have found out about the 1000 calories consistently dinner plan and need to seek after it, for the direct clarification, that you are not starving, simply diminishing the calories!

It is clear your criticalness. Being overweight is causing you ceaseless ailments and possibly you can not get any rest as you are a setback of rest apnea - a prompt exit being overweight.

To get directly to the point, there is nothing genuinely wrong with the 1000 calories consistently supper plan, on the other hand, really this is seen as a fairly unprecedented measure to get more slender.

Calorie is the energy the body needs and gets it from the food sources that we eat.

So when you decline the calorie utilization so profoundly, it ordinarily suggests that you are keeping the combination from getting key energy. Moreover, it is recommended not to choose 1000 calories day by day course of action, with the exception of on the off chance that you have the expert's gathered approve in such way and the weight decrease is immovably checked.

We consistently commit fundamental errors in judgment when eager to get more fit. Because of nonattendance of rest, you are presently low on energy levels. Would you have the option to imagine what your condition would be where you further abatement the energy commitments by picking such a gala plan?

Here are some various factors with respect to 1000 calories each day feast plan for your idea, before you decide to follow this:

Weight decrease is ordinarily postponed with this sort of dinner plan. Notwithstanding how strong your restraint is or how much constancy you have, the most major issue of a 1000 calories consistently feast plan is that you would immediately put on the shed pounds, when you stop the supper plan.

Because of the incredibly low calorie content, 1000 calories every day plan is proposed for passing use only - for about a fortnight. Weight watchers typically take up this plan either to restart weight decrease or as such a system substance.

As demonstrated by experts such serious cut in calories may not be helpful for prosperity at whatever point carried on for longer than a week or 10 days and no more.

To ensure adequate affirmation of supplements and minerals, you should reliably consolidate a multivitamin/multi supplement all the while with this supper plan.

Such dinner plans are taken up by people who are eager to shed pounds. For your circumstance, when your fundamental point is to shed pounds to manage your rest apnea issue, this may not be the right choice, with the exception of if unequivocally recommended by your essential consideration doctor.

Before you select 1000 calories every day course of action you need to review that weight decrease ends up being doubly hard for an unwanted body.

A huge reasons why such a plan isn't fruitful for weight decrease is that after some time, such an eating routine will without a doubt frustrate the body's absorption. It is typical for the body to adhere on to every calorie that you give, searching for the crucial enhancements.

Possibly a far better decision is than find a blowout plan which considers your body's specific calorie needs, the extent that your height, weight, age and for the most part infirmity. Not solely does a decent dinner plan help you with getting fit as a fiddle in a peril free way, yet leaves you with a lot of huge peacefulness also.

4. Ultimate Diet.

Is it genuine that you are looking for the Ultimate Diet Plan to help you with shedding pounds? There are such innumerable different ones out there- - It is hard to pick just one. There are Diet Plans for almost anyone - From Children, Adults, Diabetics-There are even Diets Plans for your pets. Where to unmistakable looking? You should at first talk with your essential consideration doctor about shedding pounds first. Talking with your Doctor will help you with the pressing factor you may feel when starting an eating routine.

Most overweight people don't plan their dinners. They will just stop at an economical food put and get something there instead of orchestrating what they should eat. You would not really like to give up to your longings.

You need to limit your calorie utilization - avoid desires and endeavor to get in an extensive part of action. Exercise will go far in getting your body alive and well to assist you with devouring those wealth calories. It collects muscle which burns-through calories.

Your Ultimate Diet Plan ought to involve a Well Balanced Diet, Smaller anyway more relentless meals, no greasy or high fat food sources. Eat more fiber-like Fruits and Vegetables.

You would not really like to starve yourself by cutting you your food confirmation fundamentally. This will impact your prosperity since you body isn't used to this tremendous disaster in food utilization. You need to begin eating the right kinds of food.

5. Healthy Lifestyle Easy Recipes.

These days with our clamoring lifestyle, it is getting progressively more difficult to put energy on cooking in house. More people by and by truly prefer to go to a drive-through joint, eat and leave under 30 minutes. Generally couple of people center around what they eat and whether they are taking the sum of their crucial step by step supplements and minerals. We don't zero in if we have had adequate fiber or calcium or even protein in our food. We may not comprehend what kind of oil has been used to set up the food we are eating and in as a rule we may never ask with respect to whether we are pursuing acceptable eating routines. This may be essentially because we are overlooking that shrewd counting calories is indistinguishable from a strong lifestyle and therefore an all the more exuberant living.

Shrewd eating fewer carbs doesn't infer that we change the whole of our dietary examples. In case we basically endeavor to a few the going with thoughts, we have gained some astounding headway and improved our dietary example an extraordinary arrangement. Most importantly, endeavor to cook at home more as often as possible. It may gives off an impression of being inconvenient from the outset anyway when you start cooking at home, you will get acquainted with it and like it.

Endeavor to have some basic and fast designs for great dinners helpful. keep new and moreover some frozen trimmings at home and force yourself to use them.

A few rule flavors and flavors like strait leave, rosemary, paprika, pepper and cinnamon at home and use them in your cooking experiences.

For your consistently dietary example, center nearer around the sustenance truth of each food thing. Maybe than poor sustenances, sweets and arranged food assortments, eat vegetables, dried nuts and characteristic items. Avoid trans fats and limit your step by step taking of drenched fats like cream and margarine. Use vegetable oils, for instance, canola oil for burning or high-heat cooking and moreover olive oil for servings of blended greens and low-heat cooking. For your consistently fiber, as opposed to white breads, start eating whole wheat breads. Besides, to wrap things up, eat more white meats and less red meats.

Red meats contains horrible cholesterol and over the top eating of them should be avoided. In like manner smooth fish, for instance, salmon or cod contain a part of the significant amino acids that our body can't convey.

By following these thoughts preferably you would acknowledge a superior lifestyle and become more aware of the meaning of the great counting calories.

6. The Mediterranean Food Diet.

The Mediterranean food diet has pulled in broad thought lately, yet it has honestly been around for centuries. Experts have been dependably astounded at the long future and low pace of cardiovascular disease among people of Crete, Southern Italy, Spain and France.

The regular Mediterranean eating routine includes the going with features:

1. For the most part High Fat Intake

While fat is overall the reprobate concerning prosperity and weight-related issues, Mediterranean people get as much as 40% of their calories from fats.

Not all fats are made same, clearly - and the Mediterranean eating routine focuses generally around sound monounsaturated fat sources, for instance, Olive Oil and Omega-3 Fatty Acids from fish. Animal fats like margarine, cream and fat and completely denied from the eating schedule.

2. Low Red Meat Consumption

The Mediterranean food diet is generally low in red meats, which is striking to grow cholesterol and event of coronary sickness. Mediterraneans generally pick lean meats like fish and poultry, and shockingly then consume them in low/moderate sums.

3. High Fruit, Vegetable and Carbohydrate Intake

Italy is acclaimed for its pasta and pizza, and the Mediterranean food diet is no uncommon case. Mediterraneans in like manner consume a ton of characteristic items, vegetables, nuts, beans and breads.

4. Standard Wine Consumption

There is nothing more Italian than tasting a glass of red wine with a dinner. In reality, even the American Heart Association recommends drinking with some limitation - that is, near one glass of wine a day for a woman, and two for a man.

It is acknowledged that wine can extend levels of "good" cholesterol. For the people who wish to avoid alcohol yet need the clinical benefits, grape juice is a sublime substitute.

7. My Mind Diet Plan To The Perfect Body.

Mind over issue. That is what some really like to call it. Regardless, I don't acknowledge that is the manner in which it works. God, the Infinite Mind, or the Infinite Intelligence made the whole universe from what we see as nothing. Anyway in my examination of Holy Writings, I have found that the hid universe is truly what God encourages us to be the 'reality' of things. We have had pragmatists since always talk about how this world is just a dream to reality moreover.

If we can recognize these things to be substantial, than would it not be reasonable to deduct that it is your mind that supports and keeps up the state of your body? Envision a situation where, the ideal body is actually a thought away. Sounds unreasonable doesn't it. In light of everything, it genuinely is that clear, yet nobody anytime said that fundamental is straightforward.

The current eating routine industry nets billions of dollars reliably with everyone endeavoring to get more slender. As we overall know, the brain a lot of them miss the mark. What we can't deny is, that most of these eating routine plans don't measure up to what we think coherently about the body and how it capacities to keepor lose fat weight. So how is it possible that it would be that paying little notice to these real factors, there are at this point different people who do sort out some way to truly use these tasks and lose the weight? From my perspective, it was not the eating schedule that truly did anything. It was the trim of the mind that made the weight drop.

The clarification there are new eating regimens that reliably come out is because it by and large gives the people who are hoping to lose the weight something to trust in. Exactly when a calorie counter beginnings on another program, it isn't the effects of the program that cause them to lose the heap whatever amount of the changing acknowledge plans that are happening to them. While I do agree that the change of the way wherein they eat, what they eat, and how much exercise they get has a contributing variable to how their body will change, I don't envision that is where by far most of the credit should be given. Most of what's happening occurs in the cerebrum. The eating routine simply controls the person to change their steady guidelines of lead that have chosen their body size. At the point when new guidelines of direct are set then the cerebrum tells the body the design it should take.

All of the complicated weight control plans we have all endeavored are just proposed to do one thing genuinely, to change your viewpoint. A considerable number individuals are oblivious of this, so it is imperative that we group and sell them something so they can get tied up with the acknowledge of weight decrease. In any case, if we can surrender what a critical number of us have created upbeing come clean with are of things, than we can get passed the 'mind support' as I like to call it, and go clearly to the focal point for the game plan; your cerebrum.

A year prior, I made an objective to myself around the beginning of the year to achieve ideal prosperity and wellbeing. Over the long haul I did everything. I have a long history of going on various eating regimens and undertakings myself. I have done practically all that you can consider short of anything cautious. Since I was a kid, I have reliably been something of a thick monkey. While I really have a very strong solid structure, it doesn't exculpate the extra layer of icing that covers this beefcake. In 2006, I went on intensive eating routine undertakings, took supplements in wealth, and even went through a fourth of the year getting cleansed.

Countless the latest 'normal prosperity' information was advising me concerning how the decontaminating would have an especially huge impact in my weight considering all the excess garbage I have built upin my stomach related structure reliably. Emphatically sounds possible, considering the proportion of McDonalds and BK I have had over my lifetime. In any case, resulting to achieving everything necessary scours, I didn't lose the powerful pounds that were gloated by various researchers.

I expected different weight decrease supplements during the time that had particularly confined impact. Shockingly, a long time back they seemed to work for me better than this time around. I followed calorie restricted eating routine plans, I followed eat an immense heap of protein, and I did the carb constraint stuff. All together, I wrapped up uplosing some weight, yet deficient to have a colossal impact in my pieces of clothing size.

Taking everything into account, I was setting all of my suppositions in the ventures and not getting to the wellspring of the issue, which is to me. I have actually perceived that it is in my examinations that I keep up my body size. I have perceived how when I speak with others on the web, how they will get some data about my weight, I will reliably give a type of help for it. My main is that I am working here 16 hours consistently at the PC, along these lines with no activity, I will without a doubt gain weight. Followed upwith the dream of one day not remaining here 16 hours consistently and having the alternative to climb, and skydive, and do lots of activities that I love to do, THEN the total of my weight will dropoff, considering the way that I have all that activity.

Do you see what I have done here? I have set myself upfor dissatisfaction. This single acknowledge, which I continue talking into reality basically every other day, will overcome some different undertakings I make to lose the extra pounds. It doesn't have any effect what I do, as long as I acknowledge this, I will keepmy body in about a comparative spot it has come to recognize as what it should be. For the latest year, I have watched my weight skim inside about 5lbs of 220lbs. I can lock in and bring it down to 215lbs. By then after a short time, I climbs its way back upto 225lbs. I start to put more work into it again, and I'm back to 220lbs, and so forth While I have sorted out some way to pack on some extra muscle, which clearly has an impact in the measure of this weight is fat, I really have not really done anything critical to change my overall body structure, which is beefcake with icing generally around the middle and base.

A little while back I reviewed some appeal I got from my arrangement expert as for my weight when I edified him with respect to my circumstance to make a genuinely enormous change in my development. While he gets a kick out of the opportunity to progress worshiping yourself for essentially the way in which you are, I uncovered to him that I can regardless improve. He continued to assist me with recalling my opinion about thoughts, and how if I install my cerebrum with another psychological self view, my body will roll out the fundamental improvements. This clearly is done by contemplating the image of my new body, and tending to my mind of the shape it should be. Sounds adequately direct, and clearly I gave it a powerless primer several days and subsequently gave up because my head was at this point set on all of these tasks.

Today regardless, I have arrived at the goal that there is only one source that will change my body, and that is my cerebrum. This battle ought to be taken to where the veritable foe is found. I really feel unequivocally since it is my psychological self view that is the wellspring of my weight, and that is it. I have adequately participated in my own harm I had for the longest time been itching to have a meager, thin, and solid physic. Each time I talked about my weight, I gave reason and protection to it. My cerebrum agreed with me, and continues passing on EXACTLY what I have encouraged it to pass on. In reality, one day when I have ringed away from the reassure and make some extraordinary memories I talked about I will totally lose the weight, JUST like I have told my mind I will. Regardless, there is no clarification what so ever that I should not have that today. The solitary thing ending me, can't avoid being me.

So starting today, I am uninhibitedly articulating my intends to go on a mind diet that will change my genuine body into a fit and solid structure. This will be done by dealing with my cerebrum a conventional eating routine of mental self view that reflects decisively how I need my body to be.

The cycle is in reality fundamental. I will follow the going with regiment.

Twofold every day (without a doubt at the start of the day and evening during my petitions) I will stopfor 5 minutes and get into an easygoing state. I will by then imagine my body correctly how I need it to be while repeating these words:

I'm meager, thin, lean, and strong

During that portrayal and affirmation, I will in like manner focus in on the inclination and how it feels to have my dream body. I will play like a film to me, my life pushing ahead with this new body, and see how people react to it, and how I react to it. I will hear people offering me acclaims on how I have gotten alive and well. These are some subtle yet unimaginable differences in what I am doing here appeared differently in relation to what I see various authentication refers to doing. Your mind revolves around what you exhort it. Here is an affirmation that I found from another site for example:

I will get more fit I am getting fit as a fiddle today and reliably

The maker observes the subsequent affirmation similar to even more great and incredible, yet I say both of these are trash. The principal errands a future tense by saying 'I will'. The mind will basically keepprojecting that attestation into the future, and you really 'will' keepwanting to shed pounds. Your mind works with what it is told. The other affirmation, while it does successfully communicate the present, it is zeroin

8. The Mediterranean Diet - Is It For You?

With dozens of studies supporting the same conclusion, there is no doubt that the Mediterranean diet is one of the world's healthiest eating habits. Of course this did not happen by a stroke of luck. Researchers have identified four factors that determine a healthy lifestyle. Namely, a low-fat diet, moderate to no drinking at all, increased physical activity and non-smoking.

In terms of diet, the traditional Mediterranean diet definitely has it all. Research has proven that the kinds of foods (fat burning foods) in this diet have a lot of benefits for your health. People following this diet have less chances of contracting metabolic illnesses and have less chances of getting inflamed cells which reduces the chance of getting disease as well. The same thing can be said about Parkinson's and Alzheimer's disease. Equally important is that people in this diet do live longer as well.

Apart from less chances of coronary heart disease and other similar diseases, the Mediterranean diet also lowers the chances of getting other diseases. People following this diet can rest easy knowing that they are adding improved quality, health and years to their life.

Good, Better, Best

When it comes to fats, people tend to think that these are all bad but this stigma could not get any worse. Saturated fats come from animal products while polyunsaturated fats are produced from plants, seeds and vegetable oil among others. Monounsaturated fats are considered the healthiest and ideally should be included in your diet in place of other kinds of fat.

The good news is that the Mediterranean diet revolves around this line of thinking. Of course it is by no coincidence that this is the reason for the health benefits you get from it. All this is thanks to the kind of staple foods included in all of Mediterranean cuisine. Mediterranean cuisine takes root from several countries each with its own distinct flavor. At the heart of these dishes though are certain foods that have been proven by research to be important for good health. These fat burning foods for vitality are responsible for all the benefits of the Mediterranean diet and making you feel better at the same time.

The health benefits from the Mediterranean diet all boils down to one thing. All the foods included in the diet are rich in essential vitamins and minerals that the body needs for vitality. Consuming these foods can more or less guarantee that you are getting enough of these nutrients, lose weight and become a healthier you. So, is the Mediterranean Diet for you?

9. The Mediterranean Recipes Diet Plan.

The trimmings are new. The plans are straightforward and ideal for the people who end up with brief period to set up a sound, flavorful, and new dinner for themselves and their families. It may require some venture shopping, in any case, as none of the plans use prepackaged trimmings with added substances and fillers and all that other stuff with no solid advantage aside from stacks of calories.

So precisely what is associated with the Mediterranean Recipes diet? Most of the suppers join bread (whole grain, clearly), cheddar, olive oil, natural items, nuts, grains, vegetables, a combination of greens, and vegetables. Olive oil and lemon are two crucial bits of Mediterranean cooking. Various flavors like oregano, basil, mint and type are extensively used as is garlic. The food is clear yet flawless with each exceptional surface and flavors from amazingly unassuming to generous. It is all incredibly nutritious and strong.

To begin this eating plan, there a few things to recollect:

o Your huge wellsprings of calcium should come from yogurt and extraordinary cheddar. Salad dressings can be delivered utilizing yogurt.

o Red mean should simply be eaten up on unprecedented occasion. It is pixie easy to use other ground meats, for instance, turkey to make a burger eaten with some avocado and put on a whole wheat bun or pita.

o You need to use intermittent and secretly created produce whenever possible to ensure the sound advantage of the food. Part of our shortfall of enhancements is a result of the early picking of vegetable and characteristic item crops so they can be conveyed all through the planet.

o Make the plans without any planning avoiding the use of pre-packaged trimmings. Again new is for each situation better refreshingly and tastes better too.

o Avoid sweet treats and eat normal item, which is lower in calories and higher in fiber and enhancements.

o Eat nuts like almonds, walnuts, and cashews for a strong, nutritious chomp.

o Protein sources are from heaps of fish, some poultry and vegetables. The omega-3 unsaturated fats in the fish will keep your heart and brain working at top capability. Eggs are in like manner a respectable wellspring of protein.

o All food assortments that ought to be cooked should be warmed or burned and never seared.

10. 10 Reasons Why The Mediterranean Diet Is Good For You.

Low in Saturated Fat

Specialists and nutritionists the world over all agree that an eating routine that is high in doused fat can have negative results on a person's prosperity and success. In actuality, an eating schedule that is high in inundated fat can cause a person to persevere through coronary ailment, can provoke danger and can cause a whole host of other ailments and concern.

The Mediterranean eating routine is basic because of how it is incredibly low in submerged fat. The normal person who follows the Mediterranean eating routine confirmations under eight percent of their calories from possibly hazardous inundated fat. This is basically underneath the typical of people who don't follow a Mediterranean eating schedule.

Consolidates Plentiful Amounts of Fresh Fruits and Vegetables

Another inspiration driving why the Mediterranean eating routine is valuable for you lies in the manner that the eating routine consolidates the use of a great deal of verdant food sources. No ifs, ands or buts, the eating routine encompasses more new food sources developed starting from the earliest stage some other dietary program or plan today.

New results of the dirt beneficially affect a person's prosperity and success. People who following the Mediterranean eating routine and consume liberal servings of results of the dirt consistently have a lower event of explicit ailments including dangerous development and cardiovascular hardships.

High in Whole Grains and Fiber

A benefit in the Mediterranean eating routine is found in the manner that it brings down in the pace of specific kinds of harm. One explanation that the Mediterranean eating routine cuts down the recurrence of illness is found in the manner that the eating routine is rich in whole grains and dietary fiber. Both whole grain and fiber have shown to cut down the pace of harm, including colorectal sickness.

High in Anti-Oxidants

The Mediterranean eating routine is high in adversaries of oxidants. Foes of oxidants accept an enormous part in keeping up the body - including organs, muscles and skin - in top condition. An eating routine high in foes of oxidants is acknowledged to ensure that an individual will live a more drawn out, better life.

Low in Red Meat

Since the Mediterranean eating routine is low in red meat, the eating routine game plan endeavors to diminish the proportion of "terrible cholesterol." An eating routine low in "dreadful cholesterol" decreases the event of cardiovascular affliction, hypertension and stroke.

High in Lean Meats

The Mediterranean eating routine recollects lean meats for moderate parts. The reasonable proportion of lean meats - including fish and certain fish and fish - gives a prosperity wellspring of protein and energy for a person.

Low in Dairy

The Mediterranean eating routine is low in dairy things. Honestly, an authentic adherent to the Mediterranean eating routine fuses basically no dairy things using any and all means. Any dairy that is associated with the eating routine is low fat or non fat. Since the eating routine is low in dairy, particularly oily dairy things, the eating routine desires a person to get or keep an ideal weight. Likewise, the eating routine aides in decreasing cholesterol and endeavors to prevent coronary disease.

Thwarts Disease

As referred to, one explanation that the Mediterranean eating routine is helpful for you rests in the manner that the eating routine arrangement appears to reduce the recurrence of explicit disorders including:

- heart and cardiovascular ailment

- threatening development

- diabetes

- hypertension

- diabetes

Life expectancy

The chronicled scenery of people of the Mediterranean locale shows that the Mediterranean eating routine endeavors to extend a person's life. Additionally, while endeavoring to grow a person's life, this eating routine arrangement endeavors to ensure that a person's more expanded life will be sound as well.

A Convenient Diet Program

Finally, the Mediterranean eating routine is helpful for you since it is a solace diet program. To follow the Mediterranean eating routine you don't need to buy any remarkable things or set up an exceptional and hard to manage diet plan. At whatever point used with moderate exercise, it is a unimaginable strategy to get more slender while remaining strong.

MALINA PRONTO

Made in the USA
Middletown, DE
20 July 2025

10886766R00040